FROM
BUMP
TO BABY

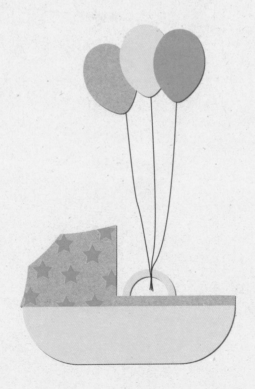

FROM BUMP TO BABY

A record book of
pregnancy and beyond

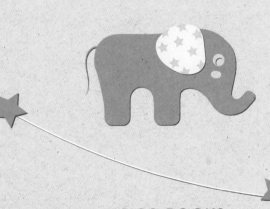

CICO BOOKS
LONDON NEW YORK

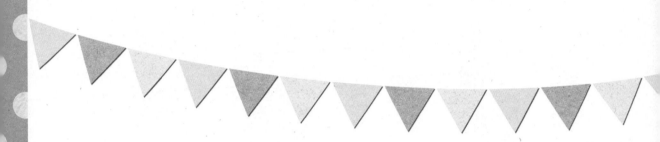

Published in 2018 by CICO Books
An imprint of Ryland Peters & Small Ltd

20–21 Jockey's Fields   341 E 116th St
London WC1R 4BW   New York, NY 10029

www.rylandpeters.com

10 9 8 7 6 5 4 3 2 1

Text, design, and illustration © CICO Books 2018

A CIP catalog record for this book is available from the Library of
Congress and the British Library.

ISBN: 978 1 78249 666 3

Printed in China

Editor: Dawn Bates

Designer: Eliana Holder

Art director: Sally Powell

Head of production: Patricia Harrington

Publishing manager: Penny Craig

Publisher: Cindy Richards

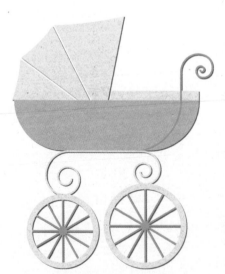

Contents

You're Pregnant!

Date You Found Out ....

Where You Were ....

Your Feelings

....

....

....

....

....

How You Told Your Partner

....

....

your partner's Reaction

....

....

....

....

PARENT(S)-TO-BE

WHO ELSE YOU TOLD

....
....
....

THEIR REACTIONS

....
....
....
....
....

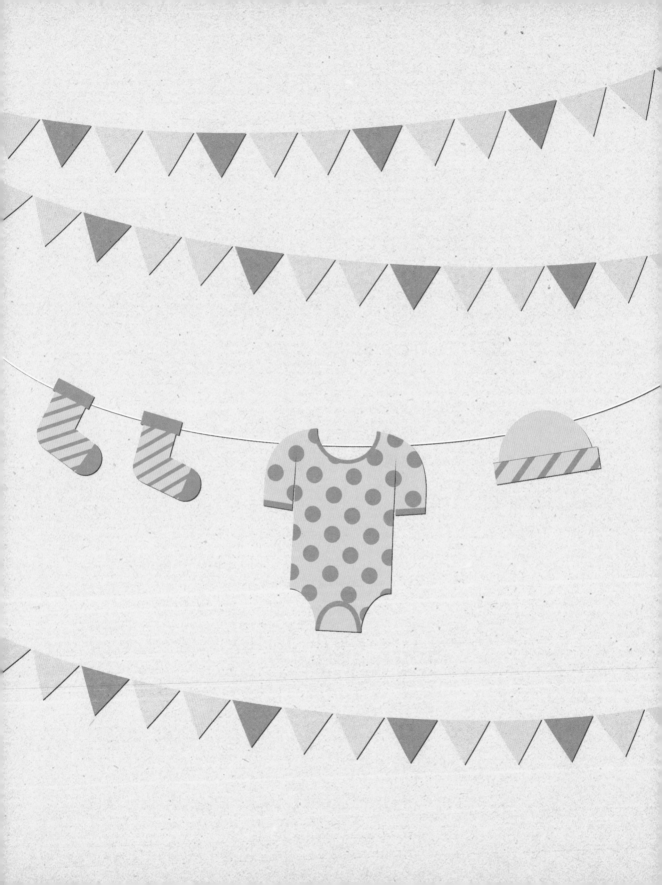

Your Pregnancy Week By Week

Keep a track of your baby's development, record how you are feeling each week, and discover some helpful pregnancy tips. There are special memories pages to fill in at the halfway and full-term stages and space, if you wish, to include photos of your precious bump.

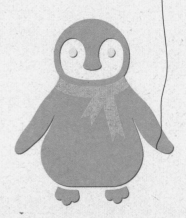

Pregnancy Calendar

January

1	2	3	4	5	6	7
8	9	10	11	12	13	14
15	16	17	18	19	20	21
22	23	24	25	26	27	28
29	30	31				

February

1	2	3	4	5	6	7
8	9	10	11	12	13	14
15	16	17	18	19	20	21
22	23	24	25	26	27	28
29						

March

1	2	3	4	5	6	7
8	9	10	11	12	13	14
15	16	17	18	19	20	21
22	23	24	25	26	27	28
29	30	31				

Use this calendar to keep a note of your hospital appointments, prenatal classes and, of course, your due date!

APRIL

1	2	3	4	5	6	7
8	9	10	11	12	13	14
15	16	17	18	19	20	21
22	23	24	25	26	27	28
29	30					

MAY

1	2	3	4	5	6	7
8	9	10	11	12	13	14
15	16	17	18	19	20	21
22	23	24	25	26	27	28
29	30	31				

JUNE

1	2	3	4	5	6	7
8	9	10	11	12	13	14
15	16	17	18	19	20	21
22	23	24	25	26	27	28
29	30					

July

1	2	3	4	5	6	7
8	9	10	11	12	13	14
15	16	17	18	19	20	21
22	23	24	25	26	27	28
29	30	31				

August

1	2	3	4	5	6	7
8	9	10	11	12	13	14
15	16	17	18	19	20	21
22	23	24	25	26	27	28
29	30	31				

September

1	2	3	4	5	6	7
8	9	10	11	12	13	14
15	16	17	18	19	20	21
22	23	24	25	26	27	28
29	30					

October

1	2	3	4	5	6	7
8	9	10	11	12	13	14
15	16	17	18	19	20	21
22	23	24	25	26	27	28
29	30	31				

November

1	2	3	4	5	6	7
8	9	10	11	12	13	14
15	16	17	18	19	20	21
22	23	24	25	26	27	28
29	30					

December

1	2	3	4	5	6	7
8	9	10	11	12	13	14
15	16	17	18	19	20	21
22	23	24	25	26	27	28
29	30	31				

WEEK 4

YOUR BABY IS ALREADY STARTING TO FORM INTERNAL ORGANS.

HOW YOU'RE FEELING THIS WEEK...

....

....

....

....

....

WEEK 5

YOUR BABY IS CHANGING SHAPE, FROM A HOLLOW CLUSTER OF CELLS TO A LONG, NARROW FORM.

HOW YOU'RE FEELING THIS WEEK...

....

....

....

....

....

WEEK 6

Your baby is about the size of the very end of your fingertip.

How you're feeling this week..

....

....

....

....

....

....

Feeling Nauseous?

Try to eat little and often, and always carry snacks with you. Rest when you can as tiredness may make your nausea worse.

WEEK 7

Your baby is starting to move, but you won't feel this for many weeks yet.

How you're feeling this week...

....

....

....

....

WEEK 8

Your baby already has elbow and knee joints!

How you're feeling this week...

....

....

....

....

WEEK 9

YOUR BABY HAS NOW LOST HER "TAIL" SO SHE LOOKS A LITTLE MORE HUMAN.

HOW YOU'RE FEELING THIS WEEK...

....

....

....

....

....

....

Skin Changes?

Hormonal changes in pregnancy may affect your skin, but it will return to normal after your baby is born. Meanwhile, try using different skincare products.

WEEK 10

YOUR BABY IS ABOUT THE SIZE OF A LARGE OLIVE.

How you're feeling this week...

....

....

....

....

....

WEEK 11

YOUR BABY IS BEGINNING TO SUCK, SWALLOW, AND YAWN.

How you're feeling this week...

....

....

....

....

....

WEEK 12

YOUR BABY IS ABOUT THE SIZE OF A LIME.

How you're feeling this week..

....

....

....

....

....

....

READY FOR YOUR FIRST SCAN?

You will be offered an ultrasound scan around now and get to see your baby for the first time! There is space on pages 52–53 for your scan photos.

WEEK 13

YOUR BABY MAY ALREADY HAVE BEGUN SUCKING HER THUMB.

How you're feeling this week..

....

....

....

....

....

WEEK 14

YOUR BABY HAS STARTED TO DEVELOP FINGERNAILS AND TOENAILS.

How you're feeling this week..

....

....

....

....

WEEK 15

YOUR BABY IS ABOUT THE SIZE OF AN APPLE.

HOW YOU'RE FEELING THIS WEEK..

....

....

....

....

....

....

....

....

HOW'S YOUR BUMP?

You may want to photograph your changing shape as your bump grows and becomes more visible. There's space on pages 26–27 and 42–43 for photos.

WEEK 16

YOUR BABY IS BECOMING MORE ACTIVE AND HE CAN NOW MAKE A FIST.

HOW YOU'RE FEELING THIS WEEK...

....

....

....

....

....

....

WEEK 17

YOUR BABY CAN ALREADY HEAR LOUD NOISES.

HOW YOU'RE FEELING THIS WEEK...

....

....

....

....

....

WEEK 18

YOUR BABY IS ABOUT THE SIZE OF A BELL PEPPER.

HOW YOU'RE FEELING THIS WEEK...

....

....

....

....

....

....

FEELING BETTER?

Hopefully the worst of your nausea has passed and you are feeling less tired. Do gentle exercise whenever you can. Seek advice from your midwife about what exercise you can do.

WEEK 19

YOUR BABY'S HEAD IS NOW ABOUT ONE-THIRD THE SIZE OF HER BODY.

HOW YOU'RE FEELING THIS WEEK..

....

....

....

....

WEEK 20

YOUR BABY IS ABOUT AS LONG AS A SMALL BANANA.

HOW YOU'RE FEELING THIS WEEK..

....

....

....

....

WEEK 21

Your baby's teeth have already developed in her gums.

How you're feeling this week...

....

....

....

....

....

....

WILL YOU FIND OUT?

Around this time, you will have another ultrasound scan and may be given the opportunity to find out the sex of your baby.

Special Memories—Halfway There

....

....

....

....

....

....

....

....

....

WEEK 22

Your baby may jump when he hears a loud noise.

How you're feeling this week...

....

....

....

....

....

WEEK 23

Your baby weighs about as much as a large mango.

How you're feeling this week...

....

....

....

....

....

WEEK 24

Your baby's facial features are now fully formed.

How you're feeling this week..

....

....

....

....

....

....

Have you made a shopping list?

You're over halfway through your pregnancy, so it may be worth budgeting and making a note of things you need to buy for your new arrival— see pages 62–63.

WEEK 25

YOUR BABY IS BEGINNING TO LOOK A LITTLE MORE ROUNDED AS SHE GAINS FAT.

How you're feeling this week...

....

....

....

....

....

WEEK 26

YOUR BABY'S NOSTRILS HAVE STARTED TO OPEN AND HE WILL BEGIN TO MAKE
BREATHING MOVEMENTS IN PREPARATION FOR DRAWING HIS FIRST BREATH.

How you're feeling this week...

....

....

....

....

....

WEEK 27

YOUR BABY NOW WEIGHS ABOUT THE SAME AS A BAG OF SUGAR (ABOUT 2.2LB/1KG).

HOW YOU'RE FEELING THIS WEEK...

....

....

....

....

....

....

....

SLEEPLESS NIGHTS?

As you begin to feel more of your baby's movements, your sleep may become disrupted. Learn the art of catnapping and do it whenever you get the opportunity.

WEEK 28

YOUR BABY IS ABOUT THE SIZE OF A BUTTERNUT SQUASH.

How you're feeling this week..

....

....

....

....

....

WEEK 29

YOUR BABY NOW HAS EYELASHES.

How you're feeling this week..

....

....

....

....

....

WEEK 30

YOUR BABY IS PASSING AROUND A PINT/HALF A LITER OF URINE EACH DAY!

How you're feeling this week...

....

....

....

....

....

....

....

Ready to Down Tools?

Make sure you have everything
in place for your maternity leave
as you'll be finishing work in
a matter of weeks.

WEEK 31

YOUR BABY'S GROWTH WILL START TO SLOW DOWN BETWEEN NOW AND HER BIRTH.

HOW YOU'RE FEELING THIS WEEK..

....

....

....

....

....

WEEK 32

YOUR BABY'S LUNGS HAVE DEVELOPED MOST OF THEIR AIRWAYS AND AIR SACS.

HOW YOU'RE FEELING THIS WEEK..

....

....

....

....

....

WEEK 33

YOUR BABY'S CHEST MOVEMENTS MAY CAUSE HER TO HICCUP OCCASIONALLY—YOU'LL FEEL THESE AS REGULAR LITTLE JUMPS.

HOW YOU'RE FEELING THIS WEEK...

....

....

....

....

....

....

....

HAVE YOU WORKED OUT A BIRTH PLAN?

Turn to pages 72–73 for things about the birth you might want to consider and decide on, such as your pain-relief options.

WEEK 34

Your baby doesn't have much room to move now—he's about 18in/46cm long, from head to heel.

How you're feeling this week..

....

....

....

....

WEEK 35

Your baby's growth will start to slow down between now and her birth.

How you're feeling this week..

....

....

....

....

WEEK 36

YOUR BABY IS LIKELY TO HAVE POSITIONED HIMSELF IN THE RIGHT POSITION, HEAD DOWN, READY FOR THE BIRTH.

HOW YOU'RE FEELING THIS WEEK...

....

....

....

....

....

....

An Urge to Nest?

It's normal to start panicking about getting your house in order before the due date. Don't overdo it though, and accept all offers of help.

WEEK 37

YOUR BABY WILL BE EXERCISING HER FACIAL MUSCLES BY FROWNING AND POUTING.

How you're feeling this week...

....

....

....

....

....

WEEK 38

YOUR AMAZING BABY HAS ALMOST LOST ALL THE FINE HAIR (LANUGO) THAT HAS COVERED HIS BODY IN THE WOMB.

How you're feeling this week...

....

....

....

....

WEEK 39

YOUR BABY'S SKULL BONES CAN OVERLAP, SO THAT HER HEAD CAN PASS THROUGH THE BIRTH CANAL WITHOUT BEING DAMAGED.

HOW YOU'RE FEELING THIS WEEK...

....

....

....

....

....

....

A Waiting Game

The days may seem long as you await your baby's arrival. Stay busy, but without venturing too far from home!

WEEK 40

YOUR BABY WILL BE BORN AROUND NOW OR, IF NOT, WITHIN THE NEXT TWO WEEKS.

HOW YOU'RE FEELING THIS WEEK...

....

....

....

....

....

....

LATE ARRIVAL

Only 3–5 percent of babies are born on their due date, so don't be surprised if your little one hasn't made an appearance yet!

Birth Announcement

Note down all the people you need to inform about the birth and whether it will be by phone, text message, or email.

Special Memories—Full Term

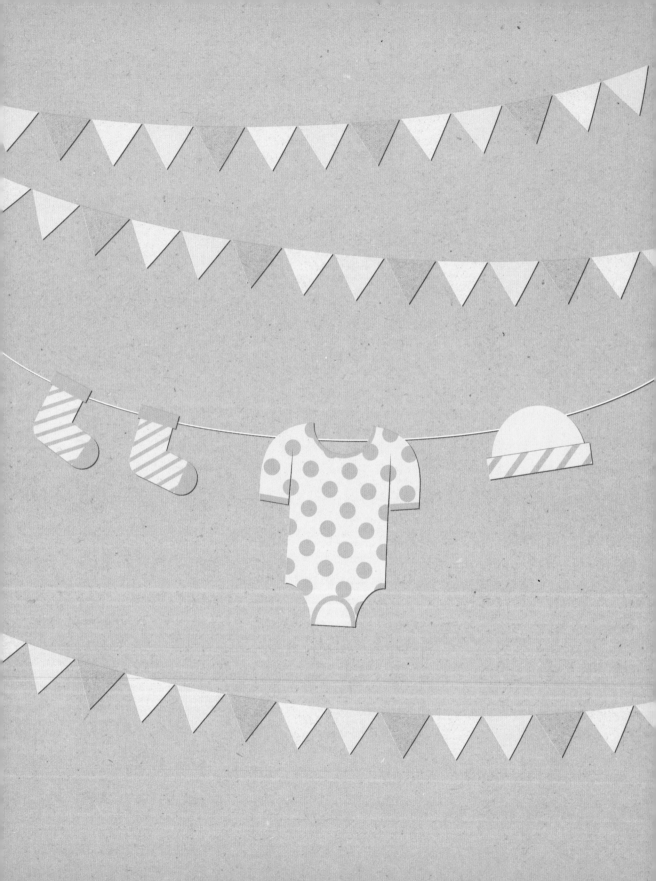

Your Medical Care

Stay on top of your healthcare with a list of important contacts, pages for your midwife appointments, including questions you might want to ask her, and space to make notes from your prenatal classes. There are special sections for your ultrasound appointments and scan photos.

Important Contacts

Midwife...Tel:...

Obstetrician...Tel:...

Hospital..Tel:...

Maternity Ward..Tel:...

Birth Partner(s)...Tel:...

....Tel:...

Other..Tel:...

....Tel:...

MEDICAL INFORMATION

Due Date...

Blood Group..

Medical Conditions

....

....

....

....

Notes

....

....

....

....

....

....

....

....

....

Prenatal Care

Your midwife will provide you with all the information you need throughout pregnancy, but before your first appointment it's worth thinking of questions you might want to ask her, such as the examples below. There's space to write notes on the page opposite and at the back of this journal.

Is the due date I've calculated correct and is it likely to change?

When will I have my first ultrasound scan?

How many ultrasound scans will I have and when?

Will I be able to find out the sex of my baby?

What prenatal tests will I be offered?

Do the tests carry any risks to me and my baby?

How often will I have prenatal appointments?

Can I contact you between appointments if I have concerns?

Do I have a choice of where to give birth?

When can I have a tour of the birthing unit?

What prenatal class options are there in my local area?

Is it safe to exercise while I'm pregnant?

Are there any foods I should avoid eating?

Should I take any supplements?

How much weight should I gain?

When will I feel my baby move and should I monitor the movements?

NOTES

MIDWIFE APPOINTMENTS

Photocopy these pages before filling them in and add them to your journal, if necessary, to build up a longer record of your appointments.

Date...

Midwife's name...

Tests carried out...

....

....

Things discussed...

....

....

Next appointment...

Date...

Midwife's name...

Tests carried out...

....

....

Things discussed...

....

....

Next appointment...

Date..

Midwife's name..

Tests carried out..

....

....

Things discussed...

....

....

Next appointment...

Notes

....

....

....

....

....

....

....

....

First Ultrasound Scan

Date..

Time..

Sonographer's name..

Who came with me..

How I felt

....

....

....

....

Second Ultrasound Scan

Date...

Time...

Sonographer's name...

Who came with me...

How I felt

....

....

....

....

....

STUDY TIME!

Prenatal classes will prepare you for the birth and for looking after your newborn baby. There's a lot of information to take in, so it's worth making notes as you go. You're likely to become good friends with the other parents-to-be at the classes as you all share this special time in your life—and you will find that they become an invaluable support network in the early weeks and months after the birth.

Name of Teacher/Midwife...

Name of Classmates

....

....

Class 1

Date...

Subjects Covered

....

....

Class 2

Date...

Subjects Covered

....

Class 3

Date...

Subjects Covered

....

Class 4

Date..

Subjects Covered

....

....

Class 5

Date..

Subjects Covered

....

....

Class 6

Date..

Subjects Covered

....

....

Class 7

Date..

Subjects Covered

....

....

Overleaf you'll find space for class notes and photos of your group.

Class Notes and Photos

You may want to take photos of you and your classmates at the beginning and end of the course, or maybe save a photo slot for all your newborns!

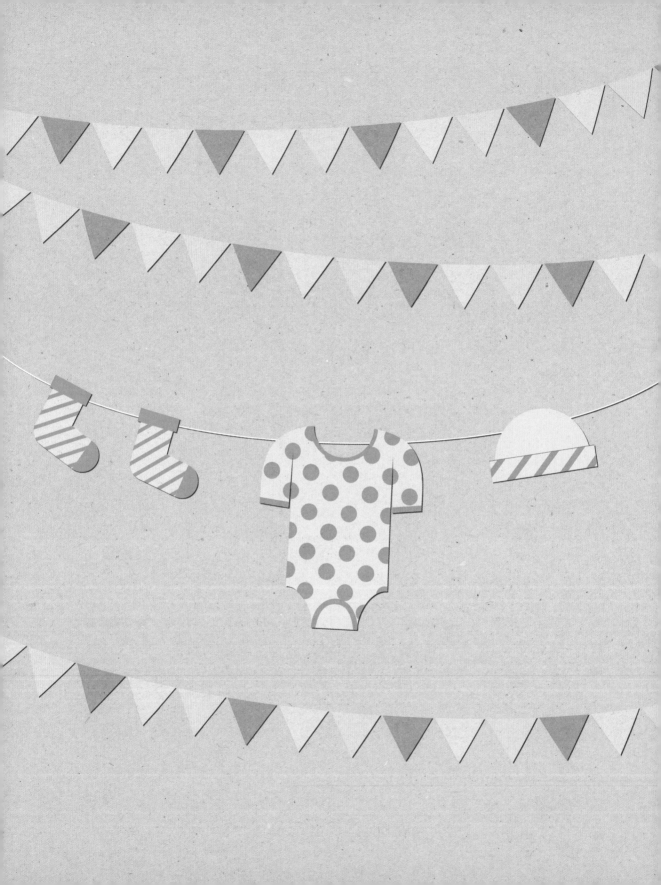

Countdown To Birth

This section will help to focus your fuzzy pregnancy brain! Use the pages to help write a birth plan, decorate the nursery, and even decide on a name. There are useful shopping checklists to ensure that you've bought everything you need for your new arrival.

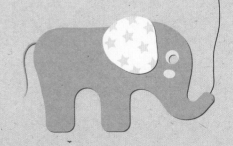

THE NAME GAME

Choosing a name for your baby can be daunting, but fun! Use the lists below to jot down those names you like and, hopefully, you can get down to at least a short-list of three that you like before the big day!

BOYS' NAMES: LONG-LIST

MEANING

1. ....

2. ....

3. ....

4. ....

5. ....

6. ....

7. ....

8. ....

9. ....

10. ....

BOYS' NAMES: SHORT-LIST

1. ....

2. ....

3. ....

Girls' Names: Long-list

1. ....
2. ....
3. ....
4. ....
5. ....
6. ....
7. ....
8. ....
9. ....
10. ....

Meaning

....
....
....
....
....
....
....
....
....
....

Girls' Names: short-list

1. ....
2. ....
3. ....

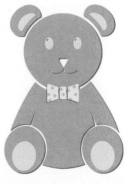

Get Ready to Shop!

Use the checklists on these pages to ensure you have bought everything you'll need for your newborn baby.

Travel

- ☐ Car seat/travel system
- ☐ Stroller that lies flat, if not part of the travel system
- ☐ Stroller accessories, such as a rain cover and/or sun shade
- ☐ Baby carrier (optional)

Sleeping

- ☐ Bassinet/Moses basket/carrycot and mattress
- ☐ Crib/cot and mattress
- ☐ Sheets and blankets
- ☐ Baby sleeping bag (optional)
- ☐ Baby monitor
- ☐ Mobile (optional)

Nappies

- ☐ Disposable diapers/nappies
- ☐ Diaper/nappy sacks
- ☐ Lotions and wipes
- ☐ Changing table and mat
- ☐ Changing bag
- ☐ Cloth diapers/Muslins

For reusable diapers/nappies, you will need liners, sterilizer, and a bucket. You may want to keep some disposables for emergencies.

Bathing

- ☐ Baby bath or bath support that can be used in the main bath
- ☐ Baby towels (optional)
- ☐ Mild baby cleanser
- ☐ Cotton wool

If you're planning to breastfeed

- ☐ Nursing bras
- ☐ Breast pads
- ☐ Nipple cream
- ☐ Breast pump (optional)

If you're planning to bottle-feed

- ☐ Sterilizer or another sterilizing method
- ☐ Bottles and brushes

Even if you're planning to breastfeed, it's handy to have this equipment from birth so that you have the option of bottle-feeding expressed breast milk.

Newborn clothes

- ☐ Onesies/Babygros (at least 8)
- ☐ Bodysuits/Vests (at least 8)
- ☐ Bibs
- ☐ Cardigans
- ☐ Socks
- ☐ Hat, depending on the season
- ☐ Coat/all-in-one suit, depending on the season
- ☐ Thermometer

Other useful equipment

- ☐ Bouncy chair
- ☐ Baby playmat
- ☐ High chair (from 6 months)

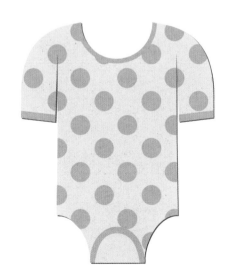
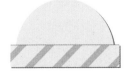
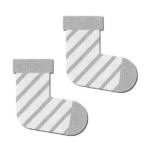

Shopping Notes

Price comparisons ....
....
....
....
....
....
....
....
....
....
....
....

Notes ....
....
....
....
....
....

Hospital Bag Checklist

Even if you're planning a home birth, it's worth packing a hospital bag a few weeks in advance of the due date in case of an emergency.

☐ Birth Plan

☐ Maternity Notes

Clothing

☐ Old T-Shirt or Nightgown

☐ Dressing Gown

☐ Thongs/Flip-Flops or Slippers

☐ Underwear

☐ Clothes to Go Home

☐ Front-opening Tops to Breastfeed

Toiletries

☐ Usual Toiletries, Plus Massage Oil and Lip Balm to Use in Labor, If You Wish, and Hair Clips/Ties For Long Hair

Snacks And Drinks

☐ Your Birth Partner Can Buy Them For You at the Hospital, But it's Worth Taking Along Things You Find Particularly Refreshing And Energizing

Items To Pass The Time

☐ Music, Magazines, Books, Tablet

Labor Accessories

☐ A Birth Ball, If Planning to Use

☐ TENS Machine, If Planning to Use

For After The Birth

☐ Nursing Bras

☐ Breast Pads

☐ Maternity Pads

For Your Newborn

☐ Nappies

☐ Cloth diapers/Muslins

☐ Onesies/Babygros and Bodysuits/Vests

☐ Socks

☐ A Going-Home Outfit, Plus Coat, Hat, and Blanket Depending On the Season

☐ Baby Car Seat

Decorating the Nursery

Favorite colors

....
....
....
....

Paint, Paper, and Fabric Notes

....
....
....
....

Furniture notes

....
....
....
....

Finishing touches

....
....
....

Stick fabric, wallpaper, and paint samples on this page.

Fabric Swatches

Wallpaper Swatches

Paint Swatches

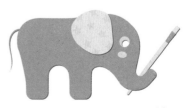

Party Time!

Having a baby shower is a wonderful opportunity to celebrate your pregnancy and impending arrival with family and friends.

Date..

Where...

Who came

....

....

....

....

What we did

....
....
....

Gifts

....
....
....
....

Invite your guests to fill in the advice pages overleaf...

Advice Pages

Ask your baby shower guests to fill in these pages. Photocopy them blank first if you want to build up an even greater record of invaluable advice!

The best advice i can give you is ....

....

....

....

....

The best advice i can give you is ....

....

....

....

....

The best advice i can give you is ....

....

....

....

....

The best advice i can give you is...
....
....
....

The best advice i can give you is...
....
....
....

The best advice i can give you is...
....
....
....

The best advice i can give you is...
....
....
....

Preparing for the Birth

Writing a birth plan is a useful way to decide on the type of labor and birth you would like, and a good way of communicating those wishes to your healthcare team. Give a copy to your birth partner(s) so that they can speak on your behalf, if necessary.

WHO WILL BE YOUR BIRTH PARTNER(S)?

HOW DO YOU FEEL ABOUT BEING INDUCED IF YOU GO PAST YOUR DUE DATE?

ARE THERE ANY LABOR POSITIONS YOU'D PARTICULARLY LIKE TO TRY?

WOULD YOU LIKE TO LABOR IN WATER IF THAT'S AN OPTION?

WHAT IS YOUR PREFERRED METHOD OF PAIN RELIEF?

How do you feel about having a Caesarean Section?

....

....

....

Does your partner want to cut the umbilical cord?

....

....

Do you want your baby passed to you straight away for
skin-to-skin contact?

....

....

Would you like to breastfeed straight away?

....

....

....

Do you want to deliver the placenta naturally?

....

....

Are there any other special requests you'd like to make known?

....

....

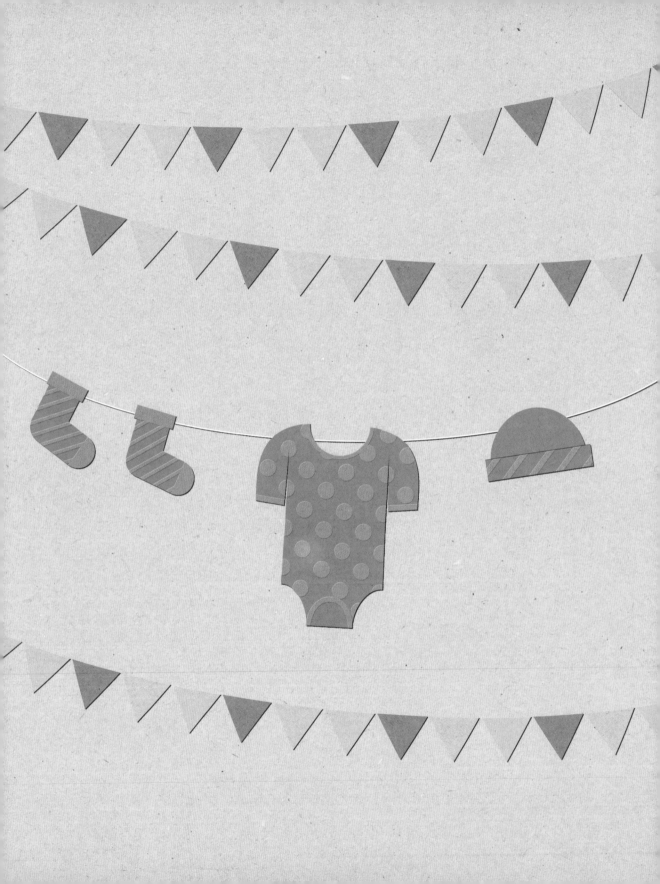

My Precious Baby

Congratulations—your beautiful newborn baby is here! Use the sleeping and feeding logs to help get your baby into a routine and note down all those special milestones as and when they happen in the coming months. Before you know it, your little one will be celebrating his or her first birthday!

WELCOME TO THE WORLD

FIRST PHOTO OF YOUR BABY

Name ....

Date of Birth ....

Time of Birth ....

Place of Birth ....

FIRST FAMILY PHOTO

Weight ....

Length..

Hair Color...

Who He/She Looked like

....

....

....

....

....

....

Sleeping Log

By keeping a record of your baby's sleep, you will see a pattern emerge and, from that, be able to establish naptime and bedtime routines. Photocopy these pages, if necessary, to build up a longer sleep record. Be aware that your baby's sleep may be affected by many things, such as growth spurts, illness, and even the weather.

Week Beginning...

	Nighttime	Morning	Afternoon	Total Sleep in 24 Hours
Monday				
Tuesday				
Wednesday				
Thursday				
Friday				
Saturday				
Sunday				

Week Beginning...

	Nighttime	Morning	Afternoon	Total Sleep in 24 Hours
Monday				
Tuesday				
Wednesday				
Thursday				
Friday				
Saturday				
Sunday				

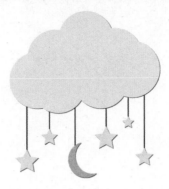

Week Beginning..

	Nighttime	Morning	Afternoon	Total Sleep in 24 Hours
Monday				
Tuesday				
Wednesday				
Thursday				
Friday				
Saturday				
Sunday				

Week Beginning..

	Nighttime	Morning	Afternoon	Total Sleep in 24 Hours
Monday				
Tuesday				
Wednesday				
Thursday				
Friday				
Saturday				
Sunday				

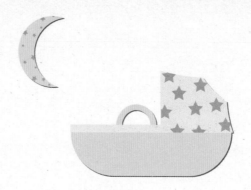

Week Beginning...

	Nighttime	Morning	Afternoon	Total Sleep in 24 Hours
Monday				
Tuesday				
Wednesday				
Thursday				
Friday				
Saturday				
Sunday				

Week Beginning...

	Nighttime	Morning	Afternoon	Total Sleep in 24 Hours
Monday				
Tuesday				
Wednesday				
Thursday				
Friday				
Saturday				
Sunday				

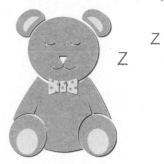

Week Beginning...

	Nighttime	Morning	Afternoon	Total Sleep in 24 Hours
Monday				
Tuesday				
Wednesday				
Thursday				
Friday				
Saturday				
Sunday				

Week beginning...

	Nighttime	Morning	Afternoon	Total Sleep in 24 Hours
Monday				
Tuesday				
Wednesday				
thursday				
Friday				
Saturday				
Sunday				

Feeding Log

In the early days, it may feel as if you are feeding all the time. Keeping a note of when and for how long your baby feeds can help you to establish some sort of routine if you want to, although you may prefer to feed on demand. There are columns for breastfeeding and bottlefeeding—you may be doing a combination of both. For breastfeeding, it can help to keep a note of which breast you fed from. Photocopy these pages, if necessary, to build up a longer feeding record.

Date	Time Fed	How Long (breast)	Amount (bottle)

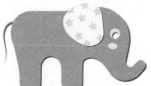

Date	Time Fed	How Long (breast)	Amount (bottle)

Date	Time Fed	How Long (breast)	Amount (bottle)

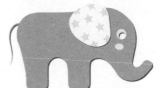

Date	Time Fed	How Long (breast)	Amount (bottle)

Precious Firsts

Date of First Bath...

Where..

Bathed by..

Date of First Outing ....

Where..

Who Came..

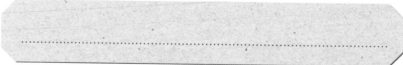

Date of First Smile ....

Who/What Made You Smile ....

First Solid Food..

Date Eaten...

Age..

....

First Crawled..

Age..

Where...

First Waved Bye-Bye...

Age..

Where...

Date First Tooth Came Through...

Age..

Which Tooth?...

First Walked..

Age..

Where...

PHOTO GALLERY

New Friends

You'll meet a lot of other parents-to-be while you're pregnant, and their children are likely to become your baby's best buddies. Use these pages to note down the names and contact details of your new social circle.

Name..

Where Met......................................

....

Due Date.......................................

Phone Number..................................

Email..

Birth Date.....................................

Baby's Name....................................

Name..

Where Met......................................

....

Due Date.......................................

Phone Number..................................

Email..

Birth Date.....................................

Baby's Name....................................

Name..

Where Met......................................

....

Due Date.......................................

Phone Number..................................

Email..

Birth Date.....................................

Baby's Name....................................

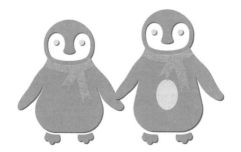

Name...

Where Met.....................................

....

Due Date.......................................

Phone Number..............................

Email..

Birth Date......................................

Baby's Name.................................

Name...

Where Met.....................................

....

Due Date.......................................

Phone Number..............................

Email..

Birth Date......................................

Baby's Name.................................

Name...

Where Met.....................................

....

Due Date.......................................

Phone Number..............................

Email..

Birth Date......................................

Baby's Name.................................

Name...

Where Met.....................................

....

Due Date.......................................

Phone Number..............................

Email..

Birth Date......................................

Baby's Name.................................

NOTES

TIME TO REFLECT

Once you feel some normality returning to your life, take the time to sit and reflect on your whole experience of pregnancy, birth, and your time with your baby so far.

....

....

....

....

....

....

....

....

....

....

....

....

....

....

....

....

....

....

....